The Red Light Therapy Handbook

Adopting Red Light For Natural Optimum Health: An Elaborately Evaluation Of The Advantages Of Red Light Therapy

GATLIN ARES

Table of Contents

Introductory 4

CHAPTER ONE 9

Gaining Knowledge Regarding Light And Its Impacts 9

The Scientific Basis For Red Light Treatment 15

Varieties Of Red Light Therapy Instruments 22

CHAPTER TWO 29

Applications For Wellness And Health 29

Red Light Therapy Implemented At Home .35

CHAPTER THREE 43

Combining Red Light Therapy WIth Additional Therapies 43

Lifestyle And Nutritional Considerations ...50

Summary 57

THE END 59

Introductory

Red Light Therapy (RLT), alternatively referred to as low-level laser therapy (LLLT) or photobiomodulation (PBM), is a type of light therapy that induces and advances diverse physiological responses within the cells of the body through the utilization of red or near-infrared light. By exposing the epidermis and body tissues to low levels of red or near-infrared light, typically via light-emitting diodes (LEDs) or low-level lasers, the treatment is accomplished.

Red light therapy commonly employs light wavelengths within the approximate range of 630 to 850 nanometers. It is postulated that cells can absorb these particular wavelengths, resulting in an assortment of physiological responses. The following are some of the purported advantages of red light therapy:

• Enhanced ATP Production: It is hypothesized that red light therapy will augment the synthesis of adenosine triphosphate (ATP), an energy-supplying molecule for cellular processes.

• Light stimulation may elicit a range of cellular responses, including enhanced mitochondrial function and the activation of particular enzymes, thereby potentially promoting cellular well-being.

• Red light therapy may assist in the improvement of blood circulation through the stimulation of new capillary formation and the enhancement of existing blood vessel function.

• Decreased Inflammation: Several research studies indicate that red light therapy might exhibit anti-inflammatory properties, thereby potentially mitigating inflammation across a range of tissues.

• Analgesic (pain-relieving) Properties: Red light therapy has the potential to alleviate pain and is therefore considered a viable treatment option for pain-related conditions.

• Red light therapy has the potential to facilitate the recovery from incisions and injuries through its ability to stimulate tissue regeneration and repair.

• Skin Health: Certain individuals employ red light therapy for aesthetic intentions, asserting that it can enhance the overall appearance of the skin, diminish wrinkles, and stimulate collagen production.

It is crucial to acknowledge that although certain conditions may be supported by some scientific evidence regarding the potential benefits of red light therapy, further investigation is required to comprehensively comprehend its mechanisms and efficacy across a range of applications.

Furthermore, it is advisable to exercise prudence when considering the utilization of red light therapy. Those who are contemplating this treatment should seek guidance from healthcare professionals, especially if they have particular medical conditions.

CHAPTER ONE
Gaining Knowledge Regarding Light And Its Impacts

An exploration of light and its effects necessitates an in-depth analysis of fundamental principles from physics, biology, and other scientific fields. A brief overview follows:

1. Spectrum of Electrons:

• Light comprises a diverse range of electromagnetic waves, including but not limited to radio waves, microwaves, infrared radiation, visible light, ultraviolet radiation, gamma rays, and X-rays.

• The visible light spectrum, which is perceptible to humans, stretches from violet to red. The wavelengths of red light are longer than those of blue or violet light.

2. The Relationship Between Wavelengths and Colors:

• An assortment of light colors are associated with distinct wavelengths. Blue light possesses lesser wavelengths in comparison to red light.

• The energy and wavelength of a photon are inversely proportional. The energy of shorter wavelengths is greater than that of longer wavelengths.

3. Photons and the Transfer of Energy:

• Light is made up of subatomic particles known as photons. Photons are capable of transferring energy to matter when they interact with it, including body cells.

• Within the realm of red light therapy, it is postulated that a multitude of cellular processes are impacted by the energy transfer from photons to cellular components.

4. Reflection and Absorption:

• An assortment of substances absorb and reflect light in distinct ways. At particular wavelengths, pigments within cells, including hemoglobin and cytochromes, absorb light.

• The selection of wavelengths in red light therapy is frequently determined by the absorption properties of chromophores, which are molecules that absorb light and are present in the target tissues.

5. Function of the Mitochondria and ATP Production:

• A potential mode of action for red light therapy entails interactions specifically with cellular structures, such as the mitochondria.

• The powerhouses of the cell, mitochondria generate adenosine triphosphate (ATP), which serves as the cells' principal energy store. Certain wavelengths of light may enhance mitochondrial function and ATP synthesis, according to a number of studies.

6. Biological Consequences:

• In the discipline of photobiology, the biological effects of light on living organisms are investigated. The investigation of the ways in which particular light wavelengths can impact cellular processes, gene expression, and a range of physiological reactions is referred to as red light therapy or photobiomodulation.

7. Clinical Therapeutic Applications:

• Red light therapy finds application in a multitude of disciplines, encompassing sports medicine, dermatology, and medicine. It is utilized for cosmetic purposes, pain management, inflammation reduction, and wound recovery.

An interdisciplinary undertaking, comprehending the impacts of light on biological systems necessitates the participation of scholars from the fields of physics, chemistry, biology, and medicine. Continuous investigation seeks to enhance our comprehension of the fundamental mechanisms that govern red light therapy and to ascertain its most effective implementations across various domains of health and wellness.

The Scientific Basis For Red Light Treatment

Red light therapy, alternatively referred to as photobiomodulation (PBM) or low-level laser therapy (LLLT), operates on the basis of the molecular and cellular interactions between light and biological tissues.

Diverse mechanisms have been postulated to elucidate the therapeutic impacts of red light therapy, although further investigation is required. The following are several pivotal components:

1. Mitochondrial Purpose:

• Red and near-infrared light particles are absorbed by mitochondria, the energy-producing organelles within cells, according to one of the central hypotheses.

• Potentially, this absorption could improve the efficiency of the electron transport chain within the mitochondria, resulting in an upregulation of adenosine triphosphate (ATP) synthesis. ATP is essential for the vitality of cells.

2. Oxidase of Cytochrome c Activation:

• It has been proposed that cytochrome c oxidase, an element of the respiratory chain within mitochondria, serves as the principal chromophore in red light therapy.

• Cytochrome c oxidase is stimulated by specific light wavelengths, which may result in enhanced cellular respiration and energy generation.

3. Nitric Oxide Emission:

• Red light therapy has the potential to induce cellular nitric oxide (NO) release. Nitric oxide is a signaling molecule that facilitates blood flow improvement via vasodilation.

• Enhanced nutrient delivery to tissues and enhanced oxygenation may be outcomes of elevated NO levels.

4. Effects Anti-Inflammatory:

• There is evidence that red light therapy decreases inflammation. It is possible that by modulating the activity of immune cells and inflammatory mediators, it can reduce pro-inflammatory signals.

5. Stimulation of factoric growth:

• Red light therapy has the potential to stimulate the secretion of growth factors, including vascular endothelial growth factor and fibroblast growth factor.

• These growth factors are involved in the processes of collagen production, angiogenesis (the formation of new blood vessels), and tissue repair.

6. Generative Expression and DNA:

• Light has the ability to affect patterns of gene expression in cells. Potential effects of red light therapy on gene expression include those associated with cellular proliferation, survival, and repair.

- The observed therapeutic effects may have been influenced by the modulation of gene expression.

7. Redox Communication:

- It is possible that red light therapy could affect redox (oxidation-reduction) signaling pathways. The equilibrium between reactive oxygen species (ROS) and antioxidant defenses within cells may be impacted.

- Regulation of reactive oxygen species (ROS) is critical for proper cellular function and signaling; red light therapy may assist in preserving this equilibrium.

8.   The   following   are neuroprotective effects:

• Several research studies have indicated that red light therapy might possess neuroprotective properties, including the ability to modulate neuroinflammation, enhance cell survival, and influence neuronal function.

It is crucial to acknowledge that although an expanding corpus of research substantiates the prospective advantages of red light therapy, the domain remains in a state of development, necessitating further investigations to comprehensively comprehend its mechanisms and optimize its implementations across diverse health conditions.

Similar to any therapeutic intervention, personalized outcomes may differ; therefore, it is advisable to seek guidance from healthcare professionals, particularly regarding particular medical issues.

Varieties Of Red Light Therapy Instruments

Red light therapy devices are available in a variety of forms, spanning from compact, portable units intended for individual use to more sizable, potent apparatuses utilized in clinical environments.

Low-level laser therapy (LLLT) devices and Light Emitting Diode (LED) devices are the two primary types of red light therapy equipment.

Here is a summary of each:

1. Red LED Light Therapy Instruments:

• Home devices are technological devices that are intended for individual use within one's residence. Frequently, they are portable, compact, and user-friendly.

• Facial Masks: Certain devices are purpose-built for facial treatments and frequently resemble face-covering masks. Utilized frequently for cosmetic objectives, they purport to provide advantages including enhanced skin pigmentation and diminished creases.

• Full-Body Panels: In order to treat more extensive areas of the body, larger LED panels or mats are utilized. These panels permit users to recline or stand in front of them for a more comprehensive treatment.

2. Devices for Low-Level Laser Therapy (LLLT):

• Handheld devices refer to compact and portable apparatuses that discharge laser light at a low intensity. They are frequently applied to specific body areas for localized treatments.

Clinical devices, including those found in wellness centers and physical therapy clinics, are characterized by their larger size and greater capacity. These devices may possess greater intensity and a greater number of features than home devices.

3. Combination apparatus:

• Certain devices integrate red light therapy with near-infrared light or other frequencies. The integration of various wavelengths has the potential to yield a more extensive spectrum of therapeutic outcomes.

• Certain devices may also include supplementary functionalities such as vibration or heat.

4. The following are targeted devices:

• Targeted devices, such as handheld devices for joint pain relief or hair growth helmets developed to address hair loss, are available for specific applications.

5. Wearable Technology:

• Wearable red light therapy devices offer a hands-free and convenient means of administering light therapy on an ongoing basis; they are specifically engineered to be worn on the body.

6. Sauna Configurations:

• In certain circles, infrared saunas, which produce infrared light containing red and near-infrared wavelengths, are categorized as a type of red light therapy. It is claimed that these saunas provide numerous health benefits, such as enhanced detoxification and circulation.

Particulars such as the intensity, treatment area coverage, wavelengths emitted, and intended application should be taken into account when selecting a red light therapy device. It is recommended to adhere to the instructions provided by the manufacturer and seek guidance from healthcare professionals when dealing with particular health conditions or concerns.

Particular responses may also be influenced by the variability in the efficacy of these devices. It is prudent, as with any health-related decision, to conduct extensive research and, if necessary, consult with healthcare professionals.

CHAPTER TWO
Applications For Wellness And Health

Red light therapy has been investigated for a range of health and wellness purposes. Although further research is required, the following areas have been suggested to have potential benefits:

1. Dermatological Health:

• Wrinkles and Aging: Red light therapy may be utilized in certain cosmetic applications to stimulate collagen production and diminish the appearance of wrinkles.

• Acne: Red light therapy may have anti-inflammatory properties and be advantageous in the treatment of acne, according to some studies.

2. Pain Administration:

• Red light therapy has garnered attention due to its potential efficacy in mitigating pain and inflammation associated with muscles and joints. This renders it a viable treatment option for a range of conditions, including arthritis, muscle strains, and joint disorders.

3. Surgical Healing:

• Wound healing may be aided by red light therapy through the stimulation of cellular regeneration and repair. Its potential applications in acute and chronic wound healing have been investigated.

4. Hair Development:

• Certain devices make claims that by stimulating hair follicles, they can increase hair volume and decrease hair loss. Frequent applications of this substance are utilized to treat conditions such as androgenetic alopecia.

5. The cognitive process:

• Red light therapy may have neuroprotective properties and may be advantageous for cognitive function, according to research. The investigation pertains to the correlation between cognitive decline and neurodegenerative diseases.

6. Mood and Resting:

• Circadian rhythms and melatonin synthesis can be impacted by light exposure, which includes red light. Certain applications investigate the potential of red light therapy to regulate temperament and enhance the quality of sleep.

7. Rehabilitation after Sports:

• Red light therapy has the potential to facilitate recuperation for athletes following strenuous physical activity. It is hypothesized that it reduces muscle fatigue and inflammation and accelerates recovery.

8. Metabolic Wellness:

• Certain studies propose that red light therapy could potentially yield favorable outcomes for metabolic parameters, including the enhancement of insulin sensitivity. This may have ramifications for diseases such as diabetes.

9. Dermatological Disorders:

• There has been research into the potential of red light therapy to treat a range of dermatological conditions, such as psoriasis and dermatitis. It potentially facilitates the regulation of inflammation and fosters the process of healing.

10. The Health of Bones:

• Current investigations are focused on the potential application of red light therapy in the enhancement of bone health and the expedited repair of fractures.

Despite the fact that evidence supports the prospective benefits of red light therapy in these areas, scientific knowledge in this regard is still developing.

Further study is required to ascertain the most effective treatment parameters and protocols for particular health conditions, as the efficacy of red light therapy may differ among individuals. It is recommended to seek guidance from healthcare professionals prior to undertaking any therapeutic intervention, particularly when it comes to addressing specific medical concerns or conditions.

Red Light Therapy Implemented At Home

Red light therapy has grown in popularity in recent years as a result of the proliferation of portable and user-friendly devices. General guidelines for the use of red light therapy at home are as follows.

1. Select the Appropriate Device:

• Choose a device for red light therapy that meets your requirements. Aspects such as the intensity, treatment area coverage, spectra emitted, and intended application should be taken into account.

2. Review the Guidelines:

• Read and adhere to the instructions provided by the manufacturer of your red light therapy device. There may be unique protocols and standards for the operation, duration, and safety of a given device.

3. Identify the Treatment Region:

• Determine which area of the body requires treatment. While some devices are intended for localized treatment, others are capable of treating complete bodies or larger areas.

4. Establish a Treatment Area:

• Select a comfortable and calm area where the red light therapy device can be utilized uninterrupted. Ensure adequate ventilation and the absence of any potential safety hazards in the area.

5. Preparing and Cleaning the Skin:

• Before proceeding, cleanse the area of treatment to eliminate any makeup, lotions, or lubricants. This facilitates the greatest possible light penetration into the epidermis.

6. Establishing Positioning:

• Adhere to the guidelines provided by the manufacturer regarding the ideal distance that should be maintained between the device and the skin. Observe the prescribed distance during the entire treatment.

7. Consistency and Recurrence:

• Commence treatment for the prescribed duration, which typically spans from a few minutes to approximately 20 minutes, contingent upon the device and intended objective. Although treatment frequency can differ, it is generally advised to attend multiple sessions per week.

8. Consistency Is Crucial:

• A sustained application of red light therapy may be necessary in order to observe discernible outcomes. Consistency with a schedule will yield the greatest results.

9. Ocular Protection:

• Certain devices produce intense light that may cause ocular discomfort. Utilize spectacles or eye protection, if included with the device, to shield your eyes throughout the treatment.

10. Exercise patience:

• The attainment of results might require a period of time, and individual reactions might differ. Maintain consistency and patience with your red light therapy regimen.

11. Seeking Advice from Healthcare Experts:

• Before beginning red light therapy at home, ensure that you have consulted with healthcare professionals regarding any specific health concerns or medical conditions you may have. This is particularly crucial if red light therapy is being incorporated into a treatment regimen for a particular health condition.

12. Surveillance for Adverse Reactions:

• It is important to monitor the skin's reaction to the treatment. Should any adverse reactions occur, including irritation or an increase in erythema, it is advised to cease use immediately and seek guidance from a healthcare professional.

Keep in mind that although red light therapy is generally regarded as safe, individual reactions may differ and it might not be appropriate for all individuals.

It is imperative to adhere to the instructions provided for the device and to consult a professional for any uncertainties regarding its suitability for your particular circumstance.

CHAPTER THREE
Combining Red Light Therapy With Additional Therapies

The integration of red light therapy with other therapeutic approaches can serve as a supplementary strategy to effectively target a range of health and wellness objectives.

Nonetheless, it is critical to exercise caution when it comes to the incorporation of therapies and, when necessary, seek the advice of healthcare experts. The following factors should be taken into account when contemplating the integration of red light therapy with other therapeutic modalities.

• Consult your healthcare provider prior to integrating red light therapy into your regimen, particularly if you have pre-existing medical conditions or are currently undergoing specific treatments. They are able to offer advice regarding the suitability of red light therapy and its potential interactions with other therapeutic modalities.

• Determine therapeutic methodologies that have the potential to enhance the advantages of red light therapy. By integrating red light therapy with physical therapy or exercise, for instance, the benefits for joint health and muscle recovery could be amplified.

• Establish unambiguous health and wellness objectives and evaluate the potential contributions of various therapies, such as red light therapy, towards their realization.

• When working with a healthcare team or multiple practitioners, transparency regarding the application of red light therapy is essential. It is imperative to inform every member of the healthcare staff regarding the therapies that are being integrated.

• The scheduling and sequence of therapies should be considered. For instance, one may opt to integrate red light therapy prior to engaging in meditation or other relaxation practices when employing it to induce relaxation and alleviate tension.

• Observe the manner in which your body reacts to the combination of treatments. Notify your healthcare provider of any unforeseen reactions or changes in your health status, and be willing to modify your approach accordingly.

• Adapt the integration of therapeutic interventions to suit particular health conditions. An instance of this would be the incorporation of red light therapy into the therapeutic regimen for specific dermatological conditions, pain management, or mood disorders.

• Determine how dietary, physical activity, and sleep patterns affect the efficacy of red light therapy in conjunction with other therapeutic modalities. A comprehensive approach to health may entail the optimization of various facets of one's lifestyle.

• Comprehend the prospective benefits and mechanisms of red light therapy. With this knowledge, you can make well-informed decisions regarding the integration of this therapy with others.

• Maintain consistent follow-up appointments with your healthcare provider in order to evaluate your progress and implement any required modifications to your treatment regimen.

• Evaluate the incorporation of therapeutic interventions in the framework of holistic health. In conjunction with other approaches supported by scientific evidence, red light therapy can contribute to a more comprehensive and integrated approach to health.

Bear in mind that individual reactions to treatments may differ, and what proves effective for one person might not resonate with another. Approaching the integration of therapies with a personalized and informed perspective is crucial, wherein one considers their particular health requirements and objectives.

Lifestyle And Nutritional Considerations

To maximize the overall benefits of red light therapy, it is essential to consider nutrition and lifestyle factors when integrating it into your health and wellness regimen. The following are some factors to bear in mind:

Regarding nutrition:

• Incorporate an antioxidant-rich diet into your routine, as this may enhance the anti-inflammatory properties of red light therapy. Antioxidants are abundant in fruits, vegetables, nuts, and grains, among other foods.

• Maintain proper hydration. Adequate hydration is vital for optimal physiological functioning and may even amplify the benefits of red light therapy.

• It is imperative to ensure adequate intake of vital nutrients that promote collagen synthesis, epidermis health, and optimal cellular operation. Vitamins C and E, zinc, and omega-3 fatty acids are all potential components.

• It is important to exercise caution when using chemicals or hygiene products that may heighten light sensitivity. It is advisable to seek guidance from your healthcare provider regarding any uncertainties you may have regarding potential interactions.

Attitude toward lifestyle:

• It is important to adhere to consistent slumber patterns. A sufficient amount of quality sleep is critical for optimal physical and mental health. Red light therapy has the potential to induce beneficial changes in circadian cycles, which could ultimately enhance the quality of sleep.

• Regular exercise should be incorporated into one's routine. Red light therapy, in conjunction with the myriad health advantages of exercise, has the potential to augment muscle recovery and overall physical welfare.

• Engage in stress management practices, including mindfulness, deep breathing exercises, and meditation. Red light therapy has the potential to alleviate tension, and its integration with stress management techniques may produce mutually reinforcing outcomes.

• It is advisable to endeavor to maintain a well-rounded lifestyle by incorporating a variety of work, leisure, and social engagements. The incorporation of red light therapy into relaxation regimens has the potential to promote both mental and emotional health.

• Although red light therapy differs from natural sunlight, maintaining a balanced exposure remains crucial. A moderate amount of natural sunlight is essential for the synthesis of vitamin D and for overall health.

• Healthcare personnel should be consulted regarding any specific health conditions or concerns in order to verify that the incorporation of red light therapy is consistent with one's comprehensive health regimen.

• Maintain routine health examinations in order to assess your overall well-being. While red light therapy may be incorporated into a comprehensive approach, it is imperative to consider and manage additional health factors.

• Tailor your approach to suit your specific requirements and objectives. It is impossible to find a universal solution; therefore, it is important to monitor the body's reaction to various dietary and lifestyle modifications.

By integrating dietary and lifestyle elements in conjunction with red light therapy, one can establish a comprehensive strategy to bolster their health and wellness objectives. It is essential to approach these factors with a customized perspective, keeping in mind your particular requirements and circumstances. Furthermore, in order to customize an integrated approach to one's health, it can be highly beneficial to seek the counsel of healthcare professionals.

Summary

A form of light therapy, red light therapy, alternatively referred to as photobiomodulation (PBM) or low-level laser therapy (LLLT), has garnered considerable interest due to its purported advantages for health and well-being.

Red light therapy has demonstrated potential as a non-invasive and potentially advantageous modality across a range of health and wellness contexts.

Constant investigation is augmenting our comprehension of its mechanisms and honing its applications. In light of the field's ongoing development, maintaining awareness and engaging in dialogue with healthcare experts will assist you in making well-informed choices regarding the incorporation of red light therapy into your holistic health and wellness regimen.

THE END